INTERMITTENT FASTING

FOR WOMAN OVER 50

The Complete Guide to Naturally Lose Weight, Increase Energy and Detox Your Body. Learn How to Slow Down Aging and Support Hormones for a Healthier Life. |2021 Edition|

© Copyright 2021 by Sheila Moore

TABLE OF CONTENTS

Legal & Disclaimer

The information contained in this book and its contents is not designed to replace or take the place of any form of medical or professional advice; and is not meant to replace the need for independent medical, financial, legal or other professional advice or services, as may be required. The content and information in this book have been provided for educational and entertainment purposes only.

The content and information contained in this book has been compiled from sources deemed reliable, and it is accurate to the best of the Author's knowledge, information and belief. However, the Author cannot guarantee its accuracy and validity and cannot be held liable for any errors and/or omissions. Further, changes are periodically made to this book as and when needed. Where appropriate and/or necessary, you must consult a professional (including but not limited to your doctor, attorney, financial advisor or such other professional advisor) before using any of the suggested remedies, techniques, or information in this book.

Upon using the contents and information contained in this book, you agree to hold harmless the Author from and against any damages, costs, and expenses, including any legal fees potentially resulting from the application of any of the information provided by this book. This

A COMPLETE INTRODUCTION TO INTERMITTENT FASTING AND ITS COUNTLESS MENTAL AND PHYSICAL BENEFITS.

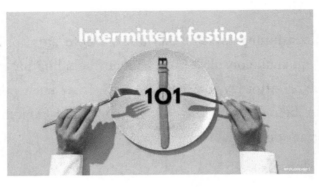

Intermittent Fasting (IF) refers to dietary eating patterns that involve not eating or severely restricting calories for a prolonged period of time. There are many different subgroups of intermittent fasting each with individual variation in the duration of the fast; some for hours, others for day(s). This has become an extremely popular topic in the science community due to all of the potential benefits on fitness and health that are being discovered.

WHAT IS INTERMITTENT FASTING (IF)?

Fasting, or periods of voluntary abstinence from food has been practiced throughout the world for ages. Intermittent fasting with the goal of improving health relatively new. Intermittent fasting involves restricting intake of food for a set/ period of time and does not include any changes to the actual foods you are eating. Currently, the most common IF protocols are a daily 16 hour fast and fasting for a whole day, one or two days per week. Intermittent fasting could be considered a natural eating pattern that humans are built to implement and it traces all the way back to our Paleolithic hunter-gatherer ancestors. The current model of a planned program of intermittent fasting could potentially help improve many aspects of health from body composition to longevity and aging. Although IF goes against the norms of our culture and common daily routine, the science may be pointing to less meal frequency and more time fasting as the optimal alternative to the normal breakfast, lunch, and dinner model. Here are two common myths that pertain to intermittent fasting.

Myth 1 - You Must Eat 3 Meals per Day: This "rule" that is common in Western society was not developed based on evidence for improved health, but was adopted as the common pattern for settlers and eventually became the norm. Not only is there a lack of scientific rationale in the 3 meal-a-day model, recent studies may be showing less meals and more fasting to be optimal for human health. One study showed that one meal a day with the same amount of daily calories is better for weight loss and body composition than 3 meals per day. This finding is a basic concept that is extrapolated into intermittent fasting and those choosing to do IF may find it best to only eat 1-2 meals per day.

Myth 2 - You Need Breakfast, its The Most Important Meal of The Day: Many false claims about the absolute need for a daily breakfast have been made. The most common claims being "breakfast increases your metabolism" and "breakfast decreases food intake later in the day".

These claims have been refuted and studied over a 16 week period with results showing that skipping breakfast did not decrease metabolism and it did not increase food intake at lunch and dinner. It is still possible to do intermittent fasting protocols while still eating breakfast, but some people find it easier to eat a late breakfast or skip it altogether and this common myth should not get in the way.

TYPES OF INTERMITTENT FASTING:

Intermittent fasting comes in various forms and each may have a specific set of unique benefits. Each form of intermittent fasting has variations in the fasting-to-eating ratio. The benefits and effectiveness of these different protocols may differ on an individual basis and it is important to determine which one is best for you. Factors that may influence which one to choose include health goals, daily schedule/routine, and current health status. The most common types of IF are alternate day fasting, time-restricted feeding, and modified fasting.

1. ALTERNATE DAY FASTING:

This approach involves alternating days of absolutely no calories (from food or beverage) with days of free feeding and eating whatever you want.

This plan has been shown to help with weight loss, improve blood cholesterol and triglyceride (fat) levels, and improve markers for inflammation in the blood.

The main downfall with this form of intermittent fasting is that it is the most difficult to stick with because of the reported hunger during fasting days.

2. MODIFIED FASTING - 5:2 DIET

Modified fasting is a protocol with programmed fasting days, but the fasting days do allow for some food intake. Generally 20-25% of normal calories are allowed to be consumed on fasting days; so if you normally consume 2000 calories on regular eating days, you would be allowed 400-500 calories on fasting days. The 5:2 part of this diet refers to the ratio of non-fasting to fasting days. So on this regimen you would eat normally for 5 consecutive days, then fast or restrict calories to 20-25% for 2 consecutive days.

This protocol is great for weight loss, body composition, and may also benefit the regulation of blood sugar, lipids, and inflammation. Studies have shown the 5:2 protocol to be effective for weight loss, improve/lower inflammation markers in the blood (3), and show signs trending improvements in insulin resistance. In animal studies, this modified fasting 5:2 diet resulted in decreased fat, decreased hunger hormones (leptin), and increased levels of a protein responsible for improvements in fat burning and blood sugar regulation (adiponectin).

The modified 5:2 fasting protocol is easy to follow and has a small number of negative side effects which included hunger, low energy, and some irritability when beginning the program. Contrary to this however, studies have also noted improvements such as reduced tension, less anger, less fatigue, improvements in self-confidence, and a more positive mood.

3. TIME-RESTRICTED FEEDING:

If you know anyone that has said they are doing intermittent fasting, odds are it is in the form of time-restricted feeding. This is a type of intermittent fasting that is used daily and it involves only consuming calories during a small portion of the day and fasting for the remainder. Daily fasting intervals in time-restricted feeding may range from 12-20 hours, with the most common method being 16/8 (fasting for 16 hours, consuming calories for 8). For this protocol the time of day is not important as long as you are fasting for a consecutive period of time and only eating in your allowed time period. For example, on a 16/8 time-restricted feeding program one person may eat their first meal at 7AM and last meal at 3PM (fast from 3PM-7AM), while another person may eat their first meal at 1PM and last meal at 9PM (fast from 9PM-1PM). This protocol is meant to be performed every day over long periods of time and is very flexible as long as you are staying within the fasting/eating window(s).

Time-Restricted feeding is one of the most easy to follow methods of intermittent fasting. Using this along with your daily work and sleep schedule may help achieve optimal metabolic function. Time-restricted feeding is a great program to follow for weight loss and body composition improvements as well as some other overall health benefits. The few human trials that were conducted noted significant reductions in weight, reductions in fasting blood glucose, and improvements in cholesterol with no changes in perceived tension, depression, anger, fatigue, or confusion. Some other preliminary results from animal studies showed time restricted feeding to protect against obesity, high insulin levels, fatty liver disease, and inflammation.

The easy application and promising results of time-restricted feeding could possibly make it an excellent option for weight loss and chronic disease prevention/management. When implementing this protocol it may be good to begin with a lower fasting-to-eating ratio like 12/12 hours and eventually work your way up to 16/8 hours.

Intermittent fasting has become a popular way to use your body's natural fat-burning ability to lose fat in a short period of time. However, many people want to know, does intermittent fasting work and how exactly does it work? When you go for an extended period of time without eating, your body changes the way that it produces hormones and enzymes, which can be beneficial for fat loss. These are the main fasting benefits and how they achieve those benefits.

Hormones form the basis of metabolic functions including the rate at which you burn fat. Growth hormone is produced by your body and promotes the breakdown of fat in the body to provide energy. When you fast for a period of time, your body starts to increase its growth hormone production. Also, fasting works to decrease the amount of insulin present in the bloodstream, ensuring that your body burns fat instead of storing it.

A short term fast that lasts 12-72 hours increases the metabolism and adrenaline levels, causing you to increase the amount of calories burned. Additionally, people who fast also achieve greater energy through increased adrenaline, helping them to not feel tired even though they are not receiving calories generally. Although you may feel as fasting should result in decreased energy, the body compensates for this, ensuring a high calorie burning regime.

Most people who eat every 3-5 hours primarily burn sugar instead of fat. Fasting for longer periods shifts your metabolism to burning fat. By the end of a 24-hour fast day, your body has used up glycogen stores in the first few hours and has spent approximately 18 of those hours burning through fat stores in the body. For anyone who is regularly active, but still struggles with fat loss, intermittent fasting can help to increase fat loss without having to ramp up a workout regime or drastically alter a diet plan.

Another benefit of intermittent fasting is that it essentially resets a person's body. Going for a day or so without eating changes a person's craving, causing them to not feel as hungry over time. If you struggle with constantly wanting food, intermittent fasting can help your body adjust to periods of not eating and help you to not feel hungry constantly. Many people notice that they begin to eat healthier and more controlled diets when they fast intermittently one day a week.

Intermittent fasting varies, but is generally recommended for about one day every week. During this day, a person may have a liquid, nutrient-filled smoothie or other low-calorie option. As the body adjusts to an intermittent fasting regime, this usually is not necessary. Intermittent fasting helps to decrease fat stores naturally in the body, by switching the metabolism to break down fat instead of sugar or muscle. It has been used by many people effectively and is an easy way to make a beneficial change. For anyone who struggles with stubborn fat and is tired of traditional dieting, intermittent fasting offers an easy and effective option for fat loss and a healthier lifestyle.

WHAT YOU CAN EXPECT

Intermittent fasting is a feeding pattern which alternates between periods of fasting and controlled eating. It is a simple dietary method divided into many types. One of the intermittent fasting methods is alternate day fasting, whereby a person takes a normal diet on particular days of the week and fasts on some. During the fasting days, one does not fully abstain from food but rather reduces calorie intake to 1/4 of the normal diet.

The other fasting type is whereby eating is restricted to a certain time window within a day. This means restricting eating between an 8 hour window eating period, which means a person eats once in every eight hours. Some people however reduce the span to either six, four or even two hours according to their convenience. The longest time that a person can stay without food on intermittent fasting is 36 hours. If practiced accordingly, it can result in a number of positive health effects.

For instance, intermittent fasting promotes general good health. It significantly reduces cravings for snack foods and sugars. The practice normalizes insulin as well as leptin sensitivity. Insulin resistance contributes to many chronic diseases such as diabetes, cancer and heart infections. Intermittent fasting will therefore protect the body from such infections.

Intermittent fasting results in improved brain health. Fasting helps the body to convert stored glycogen into glucose to release energy. If the fasting proceeds for some time, continued breakdown of body fats induces the liver to secrete ketone bodies. These small molecules are by-products of fatty acids synthesis, and the brain can use them as fuel. Research also indicates that exercise and fasting results in genes and other growth factors which are essential in recycling and rejuvenating the brain.

This type of fasting also boosts body fitness and loss of weight. Combined fasting and exercise increases effects of catalysts and cellular factors so that breakdown of glycogen and fats is maximized. Exercising while hungry therefore forces the body to burn stored fats for significant weight loss.

The program is also known to prevent cognitive decline. Research was conducted in 2006 on mice, in which water maze tests were used to assess cognitive functions of mice on normal diet and those on intermittent fasting. It was discovered that mice put on intermittent fasting experienced slower cognitive declines, which too applies to human beings.

Intermittent fasting will also boost muscle building especially in men. This is because after eating, the energy gained will be used to sustain a workout session. But if training is done while fasting, the body utilizes stored body fats to sustain the exercises. Eating after the session ensures that the energy gained is utilized in replenishing the body in the best way. This assists the muscles to quickly recover and build up.

In conclusion, intermittent fasting is a healthy practice but it could result in depression to people who cannot fully sustain it. It needs commitment and perseverance to move through the changes in diet, since only consistency will achieve these positive results.

INTERMITTENT FASTING SYSTEM

The diet you follow whilst Intermittent Fasting will be determined by the results that you are looking for and where you are starting out from as well, so take a look at yourself and ask the question what do I want from this?

If you are looking to lose a significant amount of weight then you are really going to have to take a look at your diet more closely,but if you just want to lose a few pounds for the beach then you may find that a few weeks of intermittent fasting can do that for you.

Although there are several different ways you can do intermittent fasting we are only going to look at the 24 hour fasting system which is what I used to lose 27 pounds over a 2 month period. The basic method is to fast twice a week for 24 hours, it makes sense to do this a few days apart and it is easier if you pick a day when you are busy so that you do not become distracted by feelings of hunger. Initially you may feel some hunger pangs but these will pass and as you become more accustomed to intermittent fasting you may find as I have that feelings of hunger no longer present you with a problem. You may find that you have great focus and concentration whilst fasting which is the opposite of what you would expect but many people experience this.

Whilst fasting you can and should drink plenty of water to avoid dehydration, tea and coffee are okay as long as you only take a splash of milk. If you are concerned that you are not getting enough nutrients into your body then you might consider a juice made from celery,broccoli, ginger and lime which will taste great and get some nutrient rich liquid into your body. Although if you can manage it then it would be best to stick to the water, tea and coffee.

Whatever your diet is whether its healthy or not you should see weight loss after about 3 weeks of intermittent fasting and do not be discouraged if you don't notice much progress at first, it's not a race and its better to lose weight in a linear fashion over time rather than crash losing a few pounds which you will put straight back on. After the first month you may want to take a look at your diet on non fasting days and cut out high sugar foods and any junk that you may normally eat. I have found that intermittent fasting over the long term tends to make me want to eat more healthy foods as a natural course.

If you are intermittent fasting for bodybuilding then you may want to consider looking at your macro nutrients and working out how much protein and carbohydrate you need to eat, this is much more complicated and you can find information about this on several websites which you will need to spend time researching for the best results.

There are many benefits to intermittent fasting which you will notice as you progress, some of these benefits include more energy, less bloating, a clearer mind and a general feeling of wellness. It's important not to succumb to any temptation to binge eat after a fasting period as this will negate the effect gained from the intermittent fasting period.

So in conclusion just by following a twice a week 24 hour intermittent fasting plan for a few weeks you will lose weight but if you can improve your diet on the days that you don't fast then you will lose more weight and if you can stick to this system then you will keep the weight off without resorting to any crash diets or diets that are just impossible to stick to.

INTERITTENT FASTING FOR WOMEN

For women who are interested in weight loss, intermittent fasting may seem like a great choice, but many people want to know, should women fast? Is intermittent fasting effective for women? There have been a few key studies about intermittent fasting which can help to shed some light on this interesting new dietary trend.

Intermittent fasting is also known as alternate-day fasting, although there are certainly some variations on this diet. The American Journal of Clinical Nutrition performed a study recently that enrolled 16 obese men and women on a 10-week program. On the fasting days, participants consumed food to 25% of their estimated energy needs. The rest of the time, they received dietary counseling, but were not given a specific guideline to follow during this time.

As expected, the participants lost weight due to this study, but what researchers really found interesting were some specific changes. The subjects were all still obese after just 10 weeks, but they had shown improvement in cholesterol, LDL-cholesterol, triglycerides, and systolic blood pressure. What made this an interesting find was that most people have to lose more weight than these study participants before seeing the same changes. It was a fascinating find which has spurred a great number of people to try fasting.

Intermittent fasting for women has some beneficial effects. What makes it especially important for women who are trying to lose weight is that women have a much higher fat proportion in their bodies. When trying to lose weight, the body primarily burns through carbohydrate stores with the first 6 hours and then starts to burn fat. Women who are following a healthy diet and exercise plan may be struggling with stubborn fat, but fasting is a realistic solution to this.

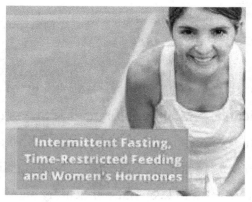

Intermittent Fasting,
Time-Restricted Feeding
and Women's Hormones

Obviously our bodies and our metabolism changes when we hit menopause. One of the biggest changes that women over 50 experience is that they have a slower metabolism and they start to put on weight. Fasting may be a good way to reverse and prevent this weight gain though. Studies have shown that this fasting pattern helps to regulate appetite and people who follow it regularly do not experience the same cravings that others do. If you're over 50 and trying to adjust to your slower metabolism, intermittent fasting can help you to avoid eating too much on a daily basis.

When you reach 50, your body also starts to develop some chronic diseases like high cholesterol and high blood pressure. Intermittent fasting has been shown to decrease both cholesterol and blood pressure, even without a great deal of weight loss. If you've started to notice your numbers rising at the doctor's office each year, you may be able to bring them back down with fasting, even without losing much weight.

Intermittent fasting may not be a great idea for every woman. Anyone with a specific health condition or who tends to be hypoglycemic should consult with a doctor. However, this new dietary trend has specific benefits for women who naturally store more fat in their bodies and may have trouble getting rid of these fat stores.

INTERMITTENT FASTING – A WAY TO LOSE WEIGHT

Health is wealth. It is described as the optimal well-being of an individual whether it is physical or psychological in nature. Staying fit and healthy promotes a positive outlook and maintains a youthful and vibrant disposition. Not only does it preserve youth, it also prolongs life. Now, one of the most innovative ways to keep oneself healthy and fit is through intermittent fasting. If you want to preserve your health, youth and the vitality of your being; then intermittent fasting should be given a try.

Intermittent fasting, as described today, is one of the cheapest fasting diets to lose weight. It doesn't require any other tools such as pills or medicines, nor does it entail any expensive gym equipment. All it simply asks is a strict and stern discipline to fasting. Intermittent fasting, by definition connotes the regulation of food intake by not ingesting anything between major meals. Also, by the word intermittent, it follows that a sequential order of eating pattern must be attained.

There's a presumption among experts that the basis on how intermittent fasting actually works can be explained by reason of anatomy and physiology; or the study of the organ and organ systems in relation to their functions within our bodies. As explained by specialists such as physicians, within our brain stem lies the seat of satiety, hunger and thirst called the hypothalamus. The hypothalamus is a complex, multifarious organ which actually orders our body when to feel the urge to gobble.

Hence, should there be any desire for man to drink or eat; the hypothalamus is the one responsible for such action. Thus, if left untrained and left to do on its own will, satiety and hunger will increase to huge proportions.

Once this happens, the urge to drink or eat will also be magnified. Of course, there is no danger or risk to eating. There is absolutely nothing wrong with that; however, the quality of the food intake we eat also determines the state of health among individuals. Likewise, if a person continually ingests foods that are not nutritious, say the one we see in fast foods or cafeterias; and done in large amounts, health is affected. Uncontrolled eating can lead to a host of diseases such as diabetes, hypertension, cardiac or heart problems and obesity.

The best way to start your fasting is to carefully plan your meals. Intermittent fasting works best if it is done regularly and habitually. This form of fasting diet to lose weight must be done in accordance with the willingness of the participant; and must be disciplined in order to achieve the desired effects. Aside from fasting, if you plan to lose weight, the amount of caloric intake must also be considered. So, aside from carefully planning the intermittent meals, the amount of calories must also be taken into consideration.

Combining the two strategies will not just make you slim; it will help you get the weight you've always wanted. Moreover, training your hypothalamus to eat intermittently will have a huge impact on your urge to eat or drink which would lead to restraining your unhealthy eating habits.

A COMPREHENSIVE GUIDE ON HOW TO CHOOSE THE FASTING METHOD THAT WILL WORK FOR YOU.

There are a few things to consider when choosing an intermittent fasting method besides thinking about which one works the best for weight loss.

Choosing an intermittent fasting method that doesn't work for you is like suffering unnecessarily and making intermittent fasting way harder than it has to be.

You might choose to fast for 20 hours a day because the weight loss results you've seen look fantastic, but you started out KNOWING you struggle to go from meal to meal without snacking.

That's a set up for failure, girl. Jumping from eating a total of 6 times a day to eating once will hurt. And it is an unnecessary hurt.

Or you choose to do a 16/8 intermittent fasting routine with most of your fasting done at night, but forget to consider that you like going on dinner dates when a fine date comes along.

As soon as that fine date shows up and ask you to dinner, you'll change your eating window. Then you find yourself barely fasting at all.

Choosing an intermittent fasting method that considers your life over if it works the best improves your chances of sticking to it.

And it's not like you have to stick with one fasting method. You can start with one for where you're at in life and your health and then transition into another routine when you're ready.

THE INTERMITTENT FASTING METHODS

16:8 Method

The 16:8 method involves having a fasting window of 16 hours and an eating window of 8 hours. Eating nothing for 16 hours and then eat 2 to 3 meals within a window of 8 hours.

INTERMITTENT FASTING 16/8

SKIP BREAKFAST
FIRST MEAL at 1 pm   LAST MEAL at 9 pm

SKIP DINNER
FIRST MEAL at 7 am   LAST MEAL at 3 pm

The 5:2 Diet

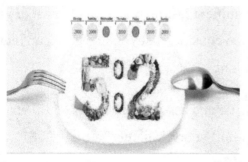

The 5:2 method involves eating normally for 5 days of the week and then eating small meals of 500 to 600 calories for 2 days of the week. For women, it's 2 meals of 250 calories each and for men it'll be 2 meals at 300 calories each.

Alternate-Day Fasting

Alternate-Day Fasting is fasting every other day. Some alternate-day fasting methods do allow for 500 calories during "fasting" days.

Eat-Stop-Eat

The Eat-Stop-Eat method involves fasting for 24 hours 1 to 2 days a week. This can be done by not eating lunch from to lunch or from dinner to dinner.

Fat Fast

Fat Fasting is consuming nothing but fat in a blended drink during a fasting window. I've seen it coupled with the 16:8 method where someone would fat fast for 16 hours in a day and then eat 2 to 3 meals within 8 hours.

Now that we've run through the different methods, let us get into how to choose the best FOR YOU.

HOW TO CHOOSE THE BEST INTERMITTENT FASTING METHOD FOR YOU BY ANSWERING 3 QUESTIONS

Choosing the best intermittent fasting routine that'll work for you is important since it'll improve your chances of sticking to it.

Trying to force an intermittent fasting method that does't work with your life and current diet is extra stress you really don't need.

Consider answering these 3 questions when determining which intermittent fasting method will work in your life and current situation with food.

How long have you been eating healthy?

Fasting tends to be the hardest when you're coming straight off the Standard American Diet due to how addictive, sugary, and high carb the diet can be.

Jumping right into a fasting window can cause sugar withdrawal symptoms that make it really difficult, and even painful to stick to.

If you're fresh off of the Standard American Diet, or tend to eat more highly processed foods than not, try starting with shorter fasting windows where most of your fast is done while you sleep.

Do this while you are transitioning to cleaner eating and detoxing from sugar.

Also cut out snacking and eat three meals of real foods during your eating window. Increase your fasting window as you adjust.

If you've been eating cleaner for some time now, and eat processed foods on occasion, you can likely get away with longer fasting windows.

If you notice it is hard to fast, eat a strict keto diet, allow your body to adapt to burning fat, and shorten your window until you feel comfortable. Then go for longer fasts.

Are you comfortable going hours or days without eating?

Some people can handle fasting an entire day while some feel more comfortable fasting for hours within a day.

Test it out for yourself. If you're comfortable going 20 hours, you might find it not too bad going a full 24. Sometimes you can fall into a 23 hour fast if you spend extra time at the gym. Pay attention to how you feel.

Struggle to fast or fear going days without eating? Pick a method that has you fasting for hours instead of a day or more.

What does your schedule look like?

Fasting is easier to do when you've got other things to do. Trust. Fasting during work, class, or while working on a project can make time less noticeable.

If you also workout, you might consider doing your fasting within windows that consist of hours instead of days. Especially when first starting out.

Working out can increase your appetite so having a fasting window that ends right after your workout instead of the following day can curve that increase and save you the torture.

Choose to fast during hours when you're the most active and if you workout, and know you still tend to deal with hunger and increased appetite, plan to end your fast afterwards.

COMMON HEALTH MYTHS AND INTERMITTENT FASTING MISCONCEPTIONS YOU NEED TO RID YOURSELF OF

Weight loss is a huge industry, it is being estimated that the US spends around 55 billion USD per year. Every Joe who knows how to run a website or post articles in a blog will look out for a pie in this huge industry, so people who wish to lose weight should not blindly follow what is being written around in the internet or what the so called experts and guru keep repeating. There is huge money to be made in this industry so invariably people will keep selling their ideas and products.

The biggest misconception, or in other words the biggest conspiracy in this industry is formulating the calorie needs for people. The calorie requirement for everyone is said to be around 2000.

Have you never seen very lean people who eat a lot and plumpy people who starve every day? The experts reason it out as the BMR (or Basal Metabolic Rate) which is not true. The bottom line is calorie sells, because of this propaganda people became highly conscious about the calorie intake, people keep checking the label for the total calories, without being aware of the other things that are not mentioned in the label.

Weight Loss or weight gain has nothing to do with calories. People become overweight, purely because they ignore the rules of nature, they fail to understand their body. Have you ever seen an overweight tiger, lion or deer? They all remain in shape because they live in accordance to the natural laws. When they hunt/ get food, they eat as much as they like, and they starve when they don't have food. When they eat, the nutrition is stored in their body, sugar is stored in the form of fat and when they starve the fat is broken down to give energy. The body consumes energy to convert glucose in to fat and also to break down fat in to energy, these metabolic activities will consume great deal of calories.

Likewise animals don't eat foods that are abnormal to seasons, the important thing is ancient Chinese medicine is not to eat food that are not in sync with the season. What we do? We eat 3 - 4 times a day and we made it as a routine. If we can keep feeding our body regularly with the calories, then what is the need of harmones like insulin and glycogon? Why should be the body perform these action of saving excessive glucose and then breakdown? Instead we can keep feeding our body what exactly is needed.

Just for this reason the ancient Indians followed fasting. When we fast regularly, unknowingly we tune the body in a particular way (The way it was created to function). Now modern researches claims a great deal health benefits and weight loss by coining new terminology for fasting like Crash Diet or IF (Intermittent Fasting). With good amount of water intake if you fast once in four days, you will get a great deal of health benefits. Your metabolic rate will get a boost, you will feel more light and energetic, here the aim is getting healthier and losing weight, losing weight is just a byproduct.

Another thing, which is being preached by everyone is about exercising and running. While they do serve the purpose, two hours of walking at a normal pace (10 miles walking) can burn just 600 calories, while good physical activity is important to be healthy, it should not be done for the sake of losing calories. The real good alternative is doing yogasanas and pranayama. When all your vital organs and glands are performing well, why should you ever worry about your weight? Your body will take care of your weight and will help you stay in shape.

The final things is being a vegetarian, it is not just important to be a vegetarian, but one should know what to eat and what not to eat, if someone claims himself to be a vegetarian and keep eating just potatoes, then there is no point in being a vegetarian.

Intermittent fasting – What it is and what it is not

When people hear the term "fasting", they often equate the term with "starving". Not eating every few hours tends to make people a little nervous. What happens if their metabolisms shut down? Won't they waste away all at once? And, when they do start eating again, everything will be stored as fat right?

Intermittent Fasting is not about starving yourself. It is simply about going without food for a short time period, then resuming your life normally. Eating like a rabbit all the time is a surefire way to fall off your diet and sabotage your goals. Eating like a rabbit part of the time, and exercising discipline and control is an effective way to improve your weight loss efforts and reach your goals.

In short, none of the above should be a real concern. Assuming an individual is healthy, meaning no underlying medical condition or disease, such as diabetes, skipping a meal or two can be an effective addition to a healthy lifestyle.

Nearly every diet that you will encounter at the book store has some sort of a trick to get the reader to eat less. Counting calories is tedious, and can be overwhelming. Reading labels and measuring ingredients can quickly take the joy out of preparing a meal. Following a recipe can be difficult enough, but to have to come up with substitutions or sacrifice entire portions of a meal to keep them within a caloric budget is undesirable for most. Such steps often lead to the abandonment of the diet altogether.

A more effective way to lose weight, or maintain weight, is to follow an intermittent fasting approach. There are several different ways to go about this. Brad Pilon of Eat Stop Eat fame advocates skipping food for an entire twenty four hour time frame. Not a bad approach, and will certainly help to reduce calories significantly so long as you don't go overboard. The downside is that an entire day of going without food is a psychological issue that some will have a hard time overcoming.

Others advocate condensing their total day's calories into a set window of anywhere from four to nine hours. Again though, this relies on counting your calories out and sticking to the plan. A smart way to go about this type of approach is to plan your meals several days in advance, so that when it's time to eat, there is no thought involved. Simply prepare the meals that have been planned, and carry on.

While both of these approaches are fine and work well for their intended purposes, a looser approach can often be a good jump off point. Many would do fine to simply skip breakfast, eat lunch a little later, and make sure that first meal is a small one. Drinking plenty of water throughout the fasted period often helps to blunt the hunger.

Skipping a meal or two, anywhere from three to five days per week should result in a net loss of anywhere between 1500-2500 calories depending on the size of the meals you are consuming. Adding that up over time comes in close to one pound per week of net caloric loss. A slightly smaller deficit can be troublesome as it will take longer to reach your goals. On the other side of this though, a smaller deficit is a more manageable deficit. The best diet is the one you can stay on.

In conclusion, it doesn't matter if you want to skip an entire day's worth of food, or one meal at a time, or count your calories and fit them in a "feeding window". The resulting reduction in calories will help to facilitate weight loss and improve your health and well being.

How intermittent fasting can help you

Intermittent fasting is a method that, if used properly, can greatly enhance your health and increase your weight loss. "Fasting" is a term used to describe a period of time when you go without eating, as is common in some religious practices. The term "intermittent" refers to the alternation of periods of eating and of fasting. So, intermittent fasting is basically a practice that involves eating within a certain time frame, and fasting in the time before and after. We all do this on a daily basis, since we are not eating when we are sleeping, but most of us do not "fast" for long enough periods of time to receive the benefits from it. Let me explain how you can alter your way of eating so that you can lose weight extremely easily without changing the types of food you eat or the amount of calories you eat.

To get the most out of intermittent fasting, you need to fast for at least 16 hours. At 16 hours and above, some of the amazing benefits of intermittent fasting kick in. An easy way to do this is to simply skip breakfast every morning. This is actually very healthy, but many people will try to tell you otherwise. By skipping breakfast, you are allowing your body to go into a caloric deficit, which will greatly increase the amount of fat you can burn and weight you can lose. Since your body is not busy digesting the food you ate, it has time to focus on burning your fat stores for energy and also for cleansing and detoxifying your body. If you find it difficult to skip breakfast, you can instead skip dinner, although I find this much more difficult. It really does not matter, but the goal is to extend the period of time you spend fasting and decrease the amount of time you spend eating. If you eat dinner at 6 o'clock at night, and don't eat until 10 the next morning, you have fasted for 16 hours. Longer is better, but you can see some pretty drastic changes from a daily 16 hour fast.

There are many ways to fast, and it is important that you choose the way that is best suited to your lifestyle so that you can stick with it and make it a lifetime habit

BEST FOOD AND DRINKS TO CONSUME WHEN YOU'RE ON THE INTERMITTENT FASTING DIET PLAN.

Of all the fad diets of the moment, intermittent fasting has garnered much attention for its convincing evidence in scientific literature. Throughout history, fasting has been utilized as an expression of political dissent, desire for spiritual reward, as well as a therapeutic tool. And it's recently gained widespread traction among fitness gurus for its touted weight loss and anti-aging effects. But that brings the big question: Is there an ultimate intermittent fasting guide so you know what to eat while you're on this diet?

First, let's take a step back and break down the basics: How does the diet work when it comes to these major intermittent fasting health benefits? Scientists postulate that the anti-aging benefits are largely due to increased insulin sensitivity, and weight loss is related to an overall reduced calorie intake because of a shortened feeding window. Simply put, when you have less time during the day to eat, you eat less. Easy, right? But a key concept, as with any diet, is determining feasibility for your lifestyle.

One study published in The Lancet Diabetes & Endocrinology showed diet-induced weight loss typically leads to a 70 percent regain in weight, so finding any type of weight-loss plan that works best for you and won't cause you any damage in the future is the key.

There are many different methods one could follow with intermittent fasting, but Andres Ayesta, MS, RDN, registered dietitian and expert in the field of fasting, says that the time-restricted feeding (TRF) approach is the best option for working adults.

"Fasting from 9 p.m. until about 1 p.m. the next day works well because most people are already skipping breakfast or are eating poor ones," Ayesta says. This approach can work well around a day job, but Ayesta also emphasizes the importance of maintaining dietary needs around this time-restricted feeding window. This means that overall diet quality and habitual food choices still matter while intermittent fasting and that you probably won't get the body of your dreams while chowing down on nothing but hamburgers and fries. In fact, eating junk food in a condensed feeding window on the IF diet may actually put you at risk of a shortfall of key nutrients such as calcium, iron, protein, and fiber, all of which are essential for normal biological function. Plus, consuming a diet rich in fruits and vegetables allows for more antioxidants in your body, which, like the metabolic effects of intermittent fasting, may contribute to a longer lifespan.

For starters, here's a breakdown of typical intermittent fasting schedules:

- Alternate Day Fasting (ADF)—1 day ad libitum eating (normal eating) alternated with 1 day of complete fasting
- Modified Alternate Day Fasting (mADF)—1 day ad libitum feeding alternated with 1 day very low-calorie diet (about 25 percent of normal caloric intake)

- 2/5—Complete fasting on 2 days of the week with 5 days ad libitum eating
- 1/6—Complete fasting on 1 day of the week with 6 days ad libitum eating
- Time Restricting Feeding (TRF)—Fasting for 12-20 hours per day (as a prolongation of the nighttime fast) on each day of the week. "Feeding window" of 4-12 hours

Here are 20 of the best foods to create the ultimate intermittent fasting food guide that will help prevent nutrient shortfalls.

1. Water

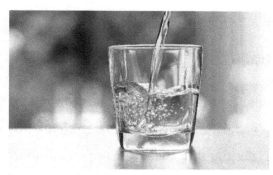

One of the most important aspects of maintaining a healthy eating pattern while intermittent fasting is to promote hydration. As we go without fuel for 12 to 16 hours, our body's preferred energy source is the sugar stored in the liver, also known as glycogen. As this energy is burned, so disappears a large volume of fluid and electrolytes. Drinking at least eight cups of water per day will prevent dehydration and also promote better blood flow, cognition, and muscle and joint support during your intermittent fasting regimen.

2. Coffee

What about a warm cup of Joe? Will a daily Starbucks run break the fast? It's a common question among newbie intermittent fasters. But worry not: Coffee is 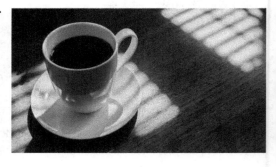 allowed. Because in its natural state coffee is a calorie-free beverage, it can even technically be consumed outside a designated feeding window. But the minute syrups, creamers, or candied flavorings are added, it can no longer be consumed during the time of the fast, so that's something to keep in mind if you usually doctor up your drink.

3. Minimally-Processed Grains

Carbohydrates are an essential part of life and are most definitely not the enemy when it comes to weight loss. Because a large chunk of your day will be spent fasting during this diet, it's important to think strategically about ways to get adequate calories while not feeling overly full. Though a healthy diet minimizes processed foods, there can be a time and place for items like whole-grain bread, bagels, and crackers, as these foods are more quickly digested for fast and easy fuel. If you intend to exercise or train regularly while intermittent fasting, these will especially be a great source of energy on the go.

4. Raspberries

Fiber, the stuff that keeps you regular was named a shortfall nutrient by the 2015-2020 Dietary Guidelines, and an article in Nutrients stated that less than 10 percent of Western populations consume adequate levels of whole fruits. With eight grams of fiber per cup, raspberries are a delicious, high-fiber fruit to keep you regular during your shortened feeding window.

5. Lentils

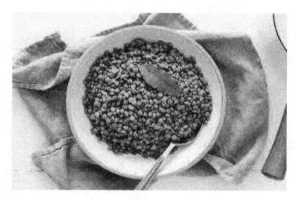

This nutritious superstar packs a high fiber punch with 32 percent of total daily fiber needs met in only half a cup. Additionally, lentils provide a good source of iron (about 15 percent of your daily needs), another nutrient of concern, especially for active females undergoing intermittent fasting.

6. Potatoes

Similar to bread, white potatoes are digested with minimal effort from the body. And if paired with a protein source, they are a perfect post-workout snack to refuel

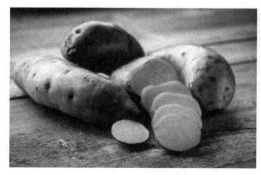

hungry muscles. Another benefit that makes potatoes an important staple for the IF diet is that once cooled, potatoes form a resistant starch primed to fuel good bacteria in your gut.

7. Seitan

The EAT-Lancet Commission recently released a report calling for a dramatic reduction in animal-based proteins for optimal health and longevity. One large study directly linked the consumption of red meat to increased mortality. Make the most of your anti-aging fast by incorporating life-extending plant-based protein substitutes like seitan. Also known as "wheat meat," this food can be battered, baked, and dipped in your favorite sauces.

8. Hummus

One of the creamiest and tastiest dips known to mankind, hummus is another excellent plant-based protein and is a great way to boost the nutritional content of staples like sandwiches, just sub it in for mayonnaise. If you're adventurous enough to make your own hummus, don't forget that the secret to the perfect recipe is garlic and tahini.

9. Wild-Caught Salmon

If your goal is to be a member of the centenarian club, you might want to read up on the Blue Zones. These five geographical regions in Europe, Latin America, Asia, and the United States are well known for dietary and lifestyle choices linked to extreme longevity. One commonly consumed food across these zones is salmon, which is high in brain-boosting omega-3 fatty acids EPA and DHA.

10. Soybeans

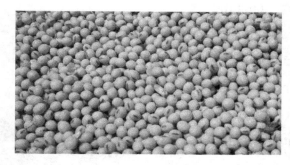 As if we needed another excuse to splurge for an appetizer at the sushi bar, isoflavones, one of the active compounds in soybeans, have demonstrated to inhibit UVB induced cell damage and promote anti-aging. So next time you host a dinner party in, impress your guests with a delicious recipe featuring soybeans.

11. Multivitamins

One of the proposed mechanisms behind why IF leads to weight loss is the fact that the individual simply has less time to eat and therefore eats less. While the principle of energy in versus energy out holds true, something that isn't often discussed is the risk of vitamin deficiencies while in a caloric deficit. Though a multivitamin is not necessary with a balanced diet of plenty of fruits and vegetables, life can get hectic, and a supplement can help fill the gaps.

12. Smoothies

If a daily supplement doesn't sound appealing, try springing for a double dose of vitamins by creating homemade smoothies packed with fruits and vegetables. Smoothies are a great way to consume multiple different foods, each uniquely packed with different essential nutrients.

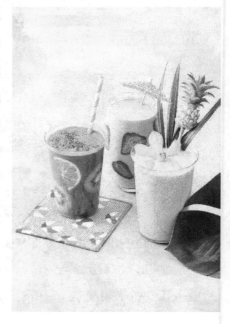

Quick tip: Buying frozen can help save money and ensure ultimate freshness.

13. Vitamin D Fortified Milk

The recommended intake of calcium for an adult is 1,000 milligrams per day, about what you'd get by drinking three cups of milk per day. With a reduced feeding window, the opportunities to drink this much might be scarce, and so it is important to prioritize high-calcium foods. Vitamin D fortified milk enhances the body's absorption of calcium and will help to keep bones strong. To boost daily calcium intake, you can add milk to smoothies or cereal, or even just drink it with meals. If you're not a fan of the beverage, non-dairy sources high in calcium include tofu and soy products, as well as leafy greens like kale.

14. Red Wine

A glass of wine and a night of beauty sleep may keep heads turning, as the polyphenol found in grapes has distinct anti-aging effects. Humans are known to have one of the enzyme classes SIRT-1, which is thought to act upon resveratrol in the presence of a caloric deficit to enhance both insulin sensitivity and longevity.

15. Blueberries

Don't let their miniature size fool you: Blueberries are proof that good things come in small packages! Studies have shown that longevity 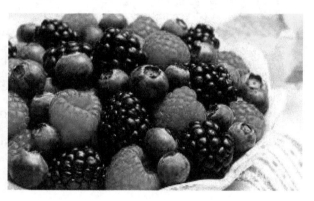 and youthfulness is a result of anti-oxidative processes. Blueberries are a great source of antioxidants and wild blueberries are even one of the highest sources of antioxidants. Antioxidants help rid the body of free radicals and prevent widespread cellular damage.

16. Papaya

During the final hours of your fast, you'll likely start to feel the effects of hunger, especially as you first start intermittent fasting. This "hanger" may, in turn, cause you to overeat in large quantities, leaving you feeling bloated and lethargic minutes later. Papaya possesses a unique enzyme called papain that acts upon proteins to break them down. Including chunks of this tropical fruit in a protein-dense meal can help ease digestion, making any bloat more manageable.

17. Nuts

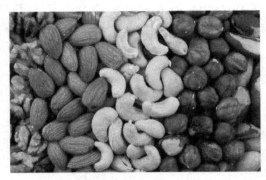 Make room on the cheese board for a mixed assortment, because nuts of all varieties are known to rid body fat and lengthen your life. A prospective trial published in the British Journal of Nutrition even associated nut consumption with a reduced risk of cardiovascular disease, Type 2 diabetes, and overall mortality.

18. Ghee

Of course, you've heard a drizzle of olive oil has major health benefits, but there are plenty of other oil options out there you can use, too. You don't want to heat an oil you're cooking with beyond its smoke point, so next time you're in the kitchen whipping up a stir-fry, consider using ghee as your oil of choice. Basically just clarified butter, it has a much higher smoke point-making, it's a great choice for hot dishes.

19. Homemade Salad Dressing

Just like your grandmother kept her cooking wholesome and simple, so should you when it comes to salad dressings and sauces. When we opt to make our own simple dressings, unwanted additives and extra sugar are avoided.

20. Branch Chain Amino Acid Supplement

A final IF-approved supplement is the BCAA. While this muscle-building aid is most beneficial for the individual who enjoys fasted cardio or hard workouts at the crack of dawn, it can be consumed all throughout the day (fasting or not) to prevent the body from going into a catabolic state and preserve lean muscle mass. Note: If you choose to follow a vegan diet pattern, this supplement may be off-limits, as most are sourced from duck feathers.

TOXIC FOODS YOU SHOULDN'T TOUCH WHILE YOU'RE FASTING INTERMITTENTLY

1. SUGAR

When people hear about drinking herbal tea, they instantly think about sweeteners. What about tea with honey? Tea with sugar?

But just because tea with honey looks the same doesn't mean it's equivalent to plain herbal tea once it's in your body. Sweetened tea is just pure simple sugars, without any fiber or fat to slow down its absorption. The result is the same as though you were to eat a handful of M&Ms: a quick spike in blood sugar, a corresponding release of insulin, and an end to the effectiveness of your fasting period. Honey does have some helpful properties, but not while fasting.

Interestingly enough, recent studies have shown that zero-calorie sweeteners can also trigger the release of insulin. This means it's also important to avoid sucralose, stevia, and artificial sweeteners while fasting. If you're really attached to your sweetened drinks, drink them during meals, not your fasting period.

2. CAFFEINE

Caffeine, found in coffee, black tea, and green tea, can also be problematic while fasting. This comes as a surprise to many people.

After all, if you're avoiding food and sugar, why not get a chemical boost to help you perk up?

Caffeine will perk you up, but the effect is temporary. Caffeine blocks the receptors for adenosine, the chemical in your body that makes you feel sleepy. But the chemicals don't go away just because caffeine is causing your body to ignore them. This means when the caffeine has worn off, you typically crash, and hard. People with a caffeine addiction know this feeling well. Combine that with a fast, and the resulting come-down can leave you unable to function.

Even folks who typically drink coffee with their breakfast can experience side effects from drinking it on an empty stomach, including physical jitters, mood swings, indigestion, and heartburn. (Sorry to say, decaf coffee isn't good for your stomach either.) Add to that the fact that many people find coffee and caffeinated tea to be bitter and unpalatable without cream, sweetener, or another additive. So if you're asking yourself, "how do I drink coffee while on a fast?" The simple answer is it's best just to leave it alone while fasting.

3. CALORIES

This should be pretty obvious, but calories can be sneaky. Bottled waters marketed towards athletes often contain calories, as do clear broths that many people consider to be water's close cousin. Chewing gum contains calories (yes, just the juice from chewing it, not even the gum itself), and bottled and packaged teas often do as well.

Vitamins and other supplements typically have some calories too; if you're fasting, leave these off until your scheduled meal. Cough drops and other medications also come with added calories. If you're sick enough to need medicine, you should probably put off fasting until you have recovered.

This doesn't mean that medicines and supplements have no place in your life if you participate in intermittent fasting. It's best, though, if you can arrange to take them with meals. Of course, if your physician has you on a strict schedule with your medicine, follow your doctor's guidelines. Staying on top of an illness is more important than any fasting routine.

BEST EXERCISES TO DO TO REMAIN HEALTHY IF YOU'RE A WOMAN OVER 50 YEARS

Want to be strong, healthy, and happy, and feel 10 years younger? Then it's time to pick up the weights. "Strength training is no longer about being buff or skinny," says trainer Holly Perkins, founder of Women's Strength Nation. "It's as critical to your health as mammograms and annual doctor visits, and it can alleviate nearly all of the health and emotional frustrations that women face today. And it becomes even more critical once you hit 50."

Age really is just a number. You might be 55, but look 40 and feel 35. Or, you might be 50, but look and feel 65. It all has to do with how well you care for your body and what you do to stay active.

When it comes to exercise, many people assume if they weren't active during their 20s, 30s or 40s, there's no point in getting started in their 50s or even later. Fortunately, that's just not true. It's never too late to start an exercise program. Starting a workout routine can help reverse some of the problems caused by inactivity and can make you feel great about yourself overall.

Let's take a close look at the benefits of exercise for women over the age of 50 and take a peek at some of the different types of exercises that will help you feel your best.

When it comes to your muscles, the saying "use 'em or lose 'em" really holds true. Starting around the age of 50, the average person loses about 1 percent of muscle each year. But the thing is, you don't have to resign yourself to losing muscle. With exercise, you can restore lost muscle, even well into your 90s.

The benefits of exercise don't stop at improving muscle mass and strength. Certain types of exercise can also help improve your bone health.

Up until about the age of 30, your body works hard to produce and build up bone. After that, you're more likely to lose bone than to create more bone. Bone loss speeds up even more during menopause because of the reduction in estrogen production. That's when the risk of osteoporosis can really set in.

But bone loss and osteoporosis aren't inevitable. Performing weight-bearing exercises, which force you to work against the forces of gravity, can help improve bone density and reduce the risk of bone breakdown.

While we're on the topic of menopause, let's take a look at some of the benefits of exercising to reduce common menopause symptoms.

The changes that happen to a woman's body during menopause, such as a decline in hormone production, can lead to weight gain and the development of excess abdominal fat. Getting or staying active while going through menopause can help you avoid some of the associated weight gain. Maintaining your weight can, in turn, help you avoid certain conditions often associated with being obese or overweight, such as Type 2 diabetes, some types of cancer and heart disease.

TYPES OF EXERCISES

Not all exercises are equal, and it's important to make sure you include a mix of different types of exercise strengthening your cardiovascular system, but also building your leg muscles. Some types of strength training exercises can also help stretch into your workout routine. The four main categories of exercise include:

> Strength training. Good weight training routines for women over 50 include lifting weights, as well as exercises that involve the use of resistance, such as Pilates or working out with resistance bands.
> Aerobic/cardiovascular. Aerobic or cardiovascular exercises are sometimes called endurance exercises, since you are supposed to maintain them for at least 10 minutes. During aerobic exercise, your heart rate and breathing should increase, but you should still be able to carry on a conversation with a workout buddy. Walking, jogging and swimming are all examples of aerobic exercise.
> Stretching. Stretching exercises help improve or maintain flexibility, reducing the risk of injury to the muscles or joints. Yoga is a popular type of stretching exercise.

> Balance. As you get older, the risk of falling increases. Exercises that help improve or maintain balance can reduce your risk of falls. A balance exercise can be as simple as standing on one foot.

Although there are four separate categories of exercise, it's important to understand exercise doesn't happen in a vacuum. For example, when you perform an aerobic exercise such as walking, you aren't just the muscles or improve your balance.

HOW MUCH EXERCISE TO GET

How much exercise should you do each week? The amount of exercise recommended for women over the age of 50 is the same as the amount recommended for other adults. Try to aim for at least 150 minutes of moderate activity or 75 minutes of vigorous activity each week. That works out to 30 minutes of exercise five days a week, or 15 minutes of vigorous exercise five days a week.

You can break up your activities into small chunks of time, but doctors recommend you devote at least 10 minutes at a time to aerobic exercise. Along with 150 or 75 minutes of activity, you should also perform strengthening exercises at least twice a week.

If you have limited mobility and have an increased risk of falling, it's also a good idea to perform balance exercises at least three days a week

GETTING THE ALL-CLEAR TO EXERCISE

Here's one crucial thing to remember before you jump into a new exercise routine, especially if you're new to working out: Get your doctor's approval before you start any new program. They can also provide guidance when it comes to the best exercises for women over 50 and the best exercises for you, based on any health concerns or issues you have.

STRENGTH TRAINING FOR 50-YEAR-OLD WOMEN

Resistance and strength training is particularly important for women aged 50 and older, as it helps slow down bone loss and can reverse the loss of muscle mass. Several workout plans for women over 50 are specifically designed to help older adults develop strength and retain muscle mass. Those programs include:

❖ Muscles in Motion - Set to music from the 1950s and '60s, Muscles in Motion helps you tighten and tone your upper and lower body, with a particular focus on the abdominal muscles. The group class uses hand weights, resistance bands and exercise balls to build strength.

❖ S.O.S - If you are particularly concerned about the risk of osteoporosis or are concerned about bone loss, S.O.S. is the fitness class for you. It focuses on resistance exercises that help improve bone health and muscle mass.

❖ SilverSneakers Classic - SilverSneakers exercise programs are available free of charge to people on Medicare. The classic program focuses on strength training as well as aerobic activities. Designed for all fitness levels, there are modifications available for people who need additional support or assistance.

STRENGTH TRAINING EXERCISES YOU CAN TRY AT HOME

1. Plank Pose - The plank can not only help strengthen and tone your core muscles, your abdominal and lower back muscles, it can also improve your balance. Planks can also help 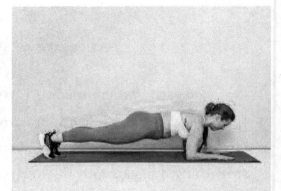 straighten your posture, which is a plus if you sit in a desk chair for much of the day.

There are a few ways to do a plank. For a high plank, get into a position as if you are at the top of a push-up, with your arms and legs straight.

Another option is a low plank, which can be easier to do if you're a beginner. Instead of supporting yourself on your hands, bend your arms at the elbow and support your weight on your forearms.

No matter which version you choose, keep your back completely straight and your head up. Your entire body should form a straight line parallel to the ground.

2. Squats With Chair - Another weight-bearing exercise that's easy to do at home is squats with a chair. During this exercise, you squat over a chair as if you were about to sit down, but don't make contact with the seat. Instead, you stand back up and repeat the process multiple times.

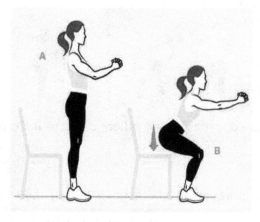

Squats not only help tone your lower body, but they can also help improve balance. When you get started, you might find it's easiest to perform the exercise with your hands and arms extended out in front of you.

3. Chest Fly - Women tend to have very weak and underdeveloped chest muscles. The chest fly is a weightlifting exercise that helps strengthen those muscles.

To do the exercise, you'll need a pair of hand weights. Lie on the floor or a mat, flat on your back, with your knees bent and your feet flat on the ground. Take one weight in each hand and raise your arms over your chest.

Slowly, open your arms out to the side, lowering your arms and wrists toward the floor but don't actually touch the ground. Keep a slight bend in your elbows, so you don't lock out your arms. Raise your arms back up and repeat.

According to a 2016 survey, nearly 40 percent of yoga practitioners in the U.S. are over the age of 50. Some women over age 50 have been 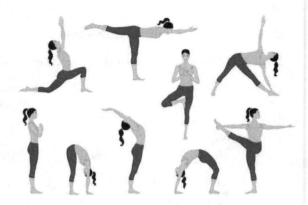 practicing yoga for years, if not decades, while others come to it for the first time in their 50s.

One thing that's important to understand about yoga is that there are many different types of styles. Some forms of yoga might be too fast-paced, strenuous or physically challenging for some people, no matter their age, while other styles are designed to be therapeutic and gentle. Unless you're an experienced yogi, it's usually best to stick with the gentler forms of yoga, which usually focus on stretching and balance more than on building strength and muscle.

Yoga Options

One of the best ways to get started with yoga and to begin an exercise program when you haven't been physically active in the past is to try chair yoga. During chair yoga, you perform many of the poses, or asanas, while seated on a chair or using a chair for support while standing. Many of our locations offer chair yoga classes.

Beginner Exercise Programs for 50-Year-Old Women

As we said, it's never too late to begin an exercise program, whether you're 50, 65 or 80. That said, if you're just starting out with physical activity, it's a good idea to look for a program designed with beginners in mind. Often, beginner exercise programs are slower-paced and feature low-impact activities, which can reduce the risk of injury.

When choosing an exercise program for beginners, look for one that combines multiple types of exercise, such as strength training with stretching and aerobic activities. That way, you'll be able to learn a variety of exercises and will get the most value from your class.

Gateway Region YMCA offers several different exercise programs for women and adults over age 50 who are looking to start a workout routine. A few of your choices include:

- SilverSneakers Cardio
- EnhanceFitness
- Fit for All

GET OUT AND EXPLORE WHILE YOU EXERCISE

Although taking an exercise class or working out at your local Y branch can be an excellent way to get fit and be social at the same time, remember you can take your workouts outside. Taking a walk around your neighborhood after dinner can be an ideal way to see what's going on around you, get some fresh air and keep your muscles strong.

You can also take things up a notch and try going for a hike on the weekends, which will give you a chance to enjoy nature while improving your endurance. When you're first getting started with hiking, take it easy. Start with short hikes on relatively flat, easy terrain. You can extend the duration of your hikes and the difficulty level as you become stronger and more confident.

MOUTH-WATERING RECIPES THAT YOU CAN TRY DURING INTERMITTENT FASTING DIET

If you don't know well the carbohydrate content of foods, your first task is to make a study of it and avoid foods high in carbohydrates such as bread, pasta, potatoes, and sugars of any kind. Carbohydrates are metabolized like sugars: like the simple sugars like those found in a soda pop. Your body is using sugars and carbohydrates as its go-to source of fuel, rather than burning the fat you are wearing around. If you deprive your body of its needed sugar, it will have no choice but to burn fat.

You push your body into fat-burning mode (ketosis) when you do not give it any sugar to burn. Ideally you will stay in this fat-burning mode for weeks and months as you drop pounds.

Here are few recipes you can try during this period.

BRUNCH RECIPES

1. Egg Scramble with Sweet Potatoes

Ingredients:

- 1 (8-oz) sweet potato, diced
- ½ cup chopped onion
- 2 tsp chopped rosemary
- Salt

- Pepper
- 4 large eggs
- 4 large egg whites
- 2 tbsp chopped chive

Directions:

Preheat the oven to 425°F. On a baking sheet, toss the sweet potato, onion, rosemary, and salt and pepper. Spray with cooking spray and roast until tender, about 20 minutes.

Meanwhile, in a medium bowl, whisk together the eggs, egg whites, and a pinch of salt and pepper. Spritz a skillet with cooking spray and scramble the eggs on medium, about 5 minutes.

Sprinkle with chopped chives and serve with the spuds.

2. Greek Chickpea Waffles

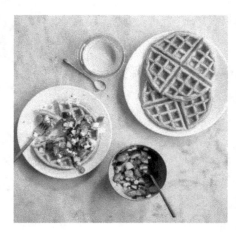

Ingredients:

- ¾ cup chickpea flour
- ½ tsp baking soda
- ½ tsp salt
- ¾ cup plain 2% Greek yogurt
- 6 large eggs
- Tomatoes, cucumbers, scallion, olive oil, parsley, yogurt, and lemon juice for serving (optional)

- Salt and pepper

Directions:

Preheat the oven to 200°F. Set a wire rack over a rimmed baking sheet and place in the oven. Heat a waffle iron per directions.

In a large bowl, whisk together the flour, baking soda, and salt. In a small bowl, whisk together the yogurt and eggs. Stir the wet ingredients into the dry ingredients.

Lightly coat the waffle iron with nonstick cooking spray. In batches, drop ¼ to ½ cup batter into each section of the iron and cook until golden brown, 4 to 5 minutes. Transfer the waffles to the oven and keep warm. Repeat with remaining batter.

Serve waffles with the savory tomato mix or a drizzle of warm nut butter and berries.

3. PB&J Overnight Oats

Ingredients:

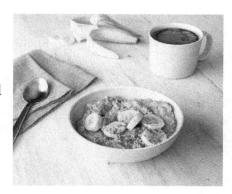

- ¼ cup quick-cooking rolled oats
- ½ cup 2 percent milk
- 3 tbsp creamy peanut butter
- ¼ cup mashed raspberries
- 3 tbsp whole raspberries

Directions:

In a medium bowl, combine oats, milk, peanut butter, and mashed raspberries. Stir until smooth.

Cover and refrigerate overnight. In the morning, uncover and top with whole raspberries.

4. Turmeric Tofu Scramble

Ingredients:

- 1 portobello mushroom
- 3 or 4 cherry tomatoes
- 1 tbsp olive oil, plus more for brushing
- Salt and pepper
- ½ block (14-oz) firm tofu
- ¼ tsp ground turmeric
- Pinch garlic powder
- ½ avocado, thinly sliced

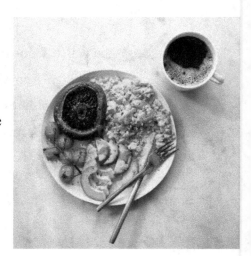

Directions:

Preheat the oven to 400°F. On a baking sheet, place the shroom and tomatoes and brush them with oil. Season with salt and pepper. Roast until tender, about 10 minutes.

Meanwhile, in a medium bowl, combine the tofu, turmeric, garlic powder, and a pinch of salt. Mash with a fork. In a large skillet over medium, heat 1 Tbsp olive oil. Add the tofu mixture and cook, stirring occasionally, until firm and egg-like, about 3 minutes.

Plate the tofu and serve with the mushroom, tomatoes, and avocado.

5. Avocado Ricotta Power Toast

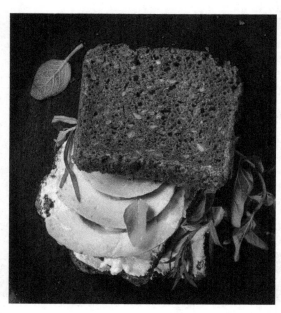

Ingredients:

- 1 slice whole-grain bread
- ¼ ripe avocado, smashed
- 2 tbsp ricotta
- Pinch crushed red pepper flakes
- Pinch flaky sea salt

Directions:

Toast the bread. Top with avocado, ricotta, crushed red pepper flakes, and sea salt. Eat with scrambled or hard-boiled eggs, plus a serving of yogurt or fruit.

6. Turkish Egg Breakfast

Ingredients:

- 2 tbsp olive oil
- ¾ cup diced red bell pepper
- ¾ cup diced eggplant
- Pinch each of salt and pepper
- 5 large eggs, lightly beaten
- ¼ tsp paprika
- Chopped cilantro, to taste
- 2 dollops plain yogurt
- 1 whole-wheat pita

Directions:

In a large nonstick skillet on medium high, heat the olive oil. Add the bell pepper, eggplant, and salt and pepper. Sauté until softened, about 7 minutes.

Stir in the eggs, paprika, and more salt and pepper to taste. Cook, stirring often, until the eggs are softly scrambled.

Sprinkle with chopped cilantro and serve with a dollop of yogurt and the pita.

7. Almond Apple Spice Muffins

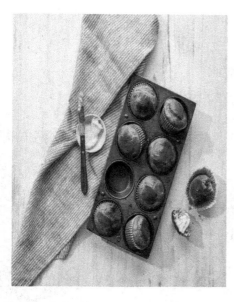

Ingredients:

- ½ stick butter
- 2 cups almond meal
- 4 scoops vanilla protein powder
- 4 large eggs
- 1 cup unsweetened applesauce
- 1 tbsp cinnamon
- 1 tsp allspice
- 1 tsp cloves
- 2 tsp baking powder

Directions:

Preheat the oven to 350°F. In a small microwave-safe bowl, melt the butter in the microwave on low heat, about 30 seconds.

In a large bowl, thoroughly mix all the remaining ingredients with the melted butter. Spray 2 muffin tins with nonstick cooking spray or use cupcake liners.

Pour the mixture into the muffin tins, making sure not to overfill (about ¾ full). This should make 10 muffins.

Place one tray in the oven and bake for 12 minutes. Make sure not to overbake, as the muffins will become too dry. When baked, remove the first tray from the oven and bake the second muffin tin the same way.

DINNER RECIPES

1. Turkey Tacos

Ingredients:

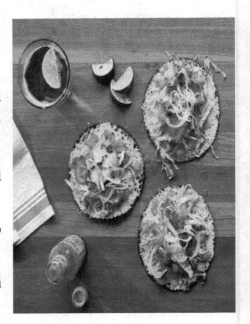

- 2 tsp oil
- 1 small red onion, chopped
- 1 clove garlic, finely chopped
- 1 lb. extra-lean ground turkey
- 1 tbsp sodium-free taco seasoning
- 8 whole-grain corn tortillas, warmed
- ¼ cup sour cream
- ½ cup shredded Mexican cheese
- 1 avocado, sliced
- Salsa, for serving
- 1 cup chopped lettuce

Directions:

In a large skillet on medium high, heat the oil. Add the onion and cook, stirring until tender, 5 to 6 minutes. Stir in the garlic and cook 1 minute.

Add the turkey and cook, breaking it up with a spoon, until nearly brown, 5 minutes. Add the taco seasoning and 1 cup water. Simmer until reduced by slightly more than half, 7 minutes.

Fill the tortillas with turkey and top with sour cream, cheese, avocado, salsa, and lettuce.

2. Healthy Spaghetti Bolognese

Ingredients:

- 1 large spaghetti squash
- 3 tbsp olive oil
- ½ tsp garlic powder
- Kosher salt and pepper
- 1 small onion, finely chopped
- 1¼ lb. ground turkey
- 4 cloves garlic, finely chopped

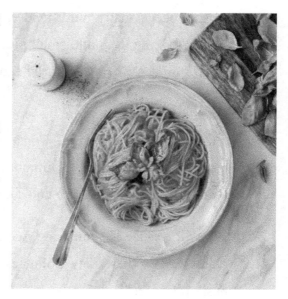

- 8 oz. small cremini mushrooms, sliced

- 3 cups fresh diced tomatoes (or 2 15-oz cans)
- 1 (8-oz) can low-sodium, no-sugar-added tomato sauce
- Fresh chopped basil

Directions:

Preheat the oven to 400°F. Cut the spaghetti squash in half lengthwise and discard seeds. Rub each half with 1/2 tbsp oil and season with garlic powder and ¼ tsp each salt and pepper. Place skin-side up on a rimmed baking sheet and roast until tender, 35 to 40 minutes. Let cool for 10 minutes.

Meanwhile, in a large skillet on medium, heat remaining 2 Tbsp oil. Add the onion, season with ¼ tsp each salt and pepper, and cook, stirring occasionally, until tender, 6 minutes. Add the turkey and cook, breaking it up into small pieces with a spoon, until browned, 6 to 7 minutes. Stir in the garlic and cook 1 minute.

Push the turkey mixture to one side of the pan, and add the mushrooms to the other. Cook, stirring occasionally, until the mushrooms are tender, 5 minutes. Mix into the turkey. Add the tomatoes and tomato sauce and simmer for 10 minutes.

While the sauce is simmering, scoop out the squash and transfer to plates. Spoon the turkey Bolognese over the top and sprinkle with basil, if desired.

3. Chicken with Fried Cauliflower Rice

Ingredients:

- 2 tbsp grapeseed oil
- 1 ¼ lb. boneless, skinless chicken breast, pounded to even thickness
- 4 large eggs, beaten
- 2 red bell peppers, finely chopped
- 2 small carrots, finely chopped
- 1 onion, finely chopped
- 2 cloves garlic, finely chopped
- 4 scallions, finely chopped, plus more for serving
- ½ cup frozen peas, thawed
- 4 cups cauliflower "rice"
- 2 tbsp low-sodium soy sauce
- 2 tsp rice vinegar
- Kosher salt and pepper

Directions:

In a large, deep skillet over medium-high, heat 1 tbsp oil. Add the chicken and cook until golden brown, 3 to 4 minutes per side. Transfer to a cutting board and let rest for 6 minutes before slicing. Add remaining 1 tbsp oil to the skillet. Add the eggs and scramble until just set, 1 to 2 minutes; transfer to a bowl.

To the skillet, add the bell pepper, carrot, and onion and cook, stirring often until just tender, 4 to 5 minutes. Stir in the garlic and cook, 1 minute. Toss with scallions and peas.

Add the cauliflower, soy sauce, rice vinegar, salt and pepper and toss to combine. Then let the cauliflower sit, without stirring, until beginning to brown, 2 to 3 minutes. Toss with the sliced chicken and eggs.

4. Sheet Pan Steak

Ingredients:

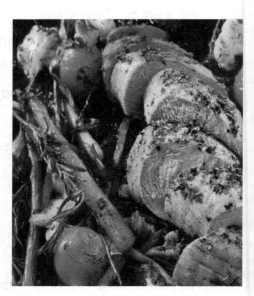

- 1 lb. small cremini mushrooms, trimmed and halved
- 1 ¼ lb. bunch broccolini, trimmed and cut into 2-in. lengths
- 4 cloves garlic, finely chopped
- 3 tbsp olive oil
- ¼ tsp red pepper flakes (or a bit more for extra kick)
- Kosher salt and pepper
- 2 1-in.-thick New York strip steaks (about 1½ lb total), trimmed of excess fat
- 1 15-oz can low-sodium cannellini beans, rinsed

Directions:

Preheat the oven to 450°F. On a large rimmed baking sheet, toss the mushrooms, broccolini, garlic, oil, red pepper flakes, and ¼ tsp each salt and pepper. Place the baking sheet in the oven and roast 15 minutes.

Push the mixture to the edges of the pan to make room for the steaks. Season the steaks with ¼ tsp each salt and pepper and place in the center of the pan. Roast the steaks to desired doneness, 5 to 7 minutes per side for medium-rare. Transfer the steaks to a cutting board and let rest 5 minutes before slicing.

Add the beans to the baking sheet and toss to combine. Roast until heated through, about 3 minutes. Serve beans and vegetables with steak.

5. Pork Tenderloin with Butternut Squash and Brussels Sprouts

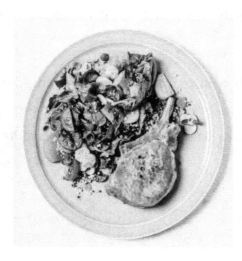

Ingredients:

- 1 ¾ lb. pork tenderloin, trimmed
- Salt
- Pepper
- 3 tbsp canola oil
- 2 sprigs fresh thyme
- 2 garlic cloves, peeled

- 4 cups Brussels sprouts, trimmed and halved
- 4 cups diced butternut squash

Directions:

Preheat the oven to 400°F. Season the tenderloin all over with salt and pepper. In a large cast-iron pan over medium high, heat 1 tbsp oil. When the oil shimmers, add the tenderloin and sear until golden brown on all sides, 8 to 12 minutes total. Transfer to a plate.

Add the thyme and garlic and remaining 2 tbsp oil to the pan and cook until aromatic, about 1 minute. Add the Brussels sprouts, the butternut squash, and a big pinch each of salt and pepper. Cook, stirring occasionally, until the vegetables are slightly browned, 4 to 6 minutes.

Place the tenderloin atop the vegetables and transfer everything to the oven. Roast until the vegetables are tender and a meat thermometer inserted into the thickest part of the tenderloin registers 140°F, 15 to 20 minutes.

Wearing oven mitts, carefully remove the pan from the oven. Allow the tenderloin to rest 5 minutes before slicing and serving with the vegetables. Toss greens with a balsamic vinaigrette to serve as a side.

6. Wild Cajun Spiced Salmon

Ingredients:

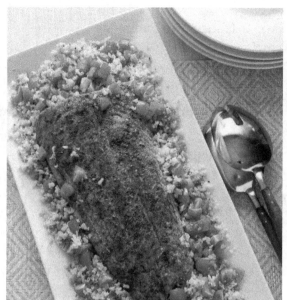

- 1½ lb. wild Alaskan salmon fillet
- Sodium-free taco seasoning
- ½ head cauliflower (about 1 lb), cut into florets
- 1 head broccoli (about 1 lb), cut into florets
- 3 tbsp olive oil
- ½ tsp garlic powder
- 4 medium tomatoes, diced

Directions:

Preheat the oven to 375°F. Place the salmon in a baking dish. In a small bowl, mix the taco seasoning with ½ cup water. Pour the mixture over the salmon and bake until opaque throughout, 12 to 15 minutes.

Meanwhile, in a food processor (in batches as necessary), pulse the cauliflower and broccoli until finely chopped and "riced."

In a large skillet on medium, heat the oil. Add the cauliflower and broccoli, sprinkle with garlic powder, and cook, tossing until just tender, 5 to 6 minutes.

Serve salmon on top of "rice" and top with tomatoes.

7. Pork Chops with Bloody Mary Tomato Salad

Ingredients:

- 2 tbsp olive oil
- 2 tbsp red wine vinegar
- 2 tsp Worcestershire sauce
- 2 tsp prepared horseradish, squeezed dry
- ½ tsp Tabasco
- ½ tsp celery seeds
- Kosher salt
- 1 pint cherry tomatoes, halved
- 2 celery stalks, very thinly sliced
- ½ small red onion, thinly sliced
- 4 small bone-in pork chops (1 in. thick, about 2¼ lb total)
- Pepper
- ¼ cup finely chopped flat-leaf parsley
- 1 small head green-leaf lettuce, leaves torn

Directions:

Heat grill to medium high. In a large bowl, whisk together the oil, vinegar, Worcestershire sauce, horseradish, Tabasco, celery seeds, and ¼ tsp salt. Toss with the tomatoes, celery, and onion.

Season the pork chops with ½ tsp each salt and pepper and grill until golden brown and just cooked through, 5 to 7 minutes per side.

Fold the parsley into the tomatoes and serve over pork and greens. Eat with mashed cauliflower or potatoes.

THE INS AND OUTS OF THE DIFFERENT APPROACHES THROUGH WHICH YOU CAN FOLLOW INTERMITTENT FASTING, INCLUDING HOW TO FOLLOW EACH FASTING PROTOCOL

Intermittent fasting weight loss is one of the most effective ways to shed off your extra pounds. The ideas on intermittent fasting weight loss challenge most of the previously held beliefs on losing. Those who are seeking new ways to lose weight effectively have quickly embraced its ideas.

WHAT IS INTERMITTENT FASTING WEIGHT LOSS?

Let me start by clarifying that intermittent fasting is not a diet. You are probably tired of trying anything with the word 'diet' on it when it comes to weight loss. Intermittent fasting is a way of eating that involves a structured program on the times when you eat and when you do not eat. You structure your program according to your fancy. If you can handle it, fast for a whole day! I recommend that you fast for 12 full hours before eating a meal. You can increase your fasting period later as you continue with the program.

What Makes it Different?

If you have tried to lose weight, you probably have tried diets such as Atkins diet based on the frequent feeding theory. Simply, proponents of such diets told you to eat often during the day. The idea was that the more you eat, the faster your metabolism. The faster your metabolism, the more fat you will lose. Of course, you do know that the more you ate, the more you wanted to eat and the more your weight remained. When you are on an intermittent program, you will have to cut down your meal frequency. Sometimes, you have to do without breakfast.

Tell Me More

You probably sleep for around 6 to 8 hours. During this time, your body is in fasting mode. When your body is in fasting mode, it usually produces more insulin. More insulin in your body causes your body to have increased insulin sensitivity. When your body has increased insulin sensitivity, you lose more fat. The brilliance of intermittent fasting weight loss program is that you skip breakfast to extend the period of your body's insulin sensitivity. This means that your body is going to be on fat loss mode for a longer period. You will lose more weight.

A longer fasting mode also has a good effect on the Growth hormone levels in your body. By skipping breakfast or eating during a specific period, your body produces Growth hormone. Growth hormone is what you want your body producing when you are trying to lose weight. This is simply because Growth hormone promotes weight loss in your body. When you are on an intermittent fasting weight loss program, your Growth hormone levels are usually at their peak. You will be losing more weight during this period. High Growth hormone levels in your body also have several other health benefits. This program is simply amazing!

Conclusion

Intermittent fasting weight loss program is radically different from most weight loss programs being promoted in the market. However, its ideas are scientifically sound when it comes to losing weight. You should give this program a go if you are serious about weight loss.

INTERMITTENT FASTING HAS MANY BENEFITS

Intermittent fasting is not so much a diet but a pattern or timing of how to eat. It is how early mankind fed itself for millennia. It has many benefits to improve our health. This article discusses intermittent fasting (IF), types of intermittent fasting and subsequent health benefits.

To be very clear this article is meant for general purposes and should not be utilized individually, but in consultation with one's health care provider.

Let's begin with stating that intermittent fasting means NO SNACKS! Snacking is out. Intermittent means we will wait an interval of time between meals.

There are various patterns that can be used for intermittent fasting. One of the simplest is: 3 square meals a day. This is a time-honored custom for many in the boomer generation and previous generations. It involves having breakfast, lunch and dinner and not eating overnight. Typically, a 4-5 hour time span between meals occurs. Since each meal is substantial the individual doesn't become hungry.

Another method of IF is to utilize the 3 square meals a day and to add a 24- 48 hour fasting time once a month where one only drinks water and sparingly drinks a vegetable broth.

There are a number of other patterns that can be pursued and are readily investigated by consulting an expert of nutrition and online references.

The benefits of IF are numerous, ranging from weight loss, improved metabolism, decreased chronic pain and lower risk of cancer.

Weight loss occurs when we refrain from eating for longer periods. If we eat frequently, we are constantly burning calories from the food we've consumed. However, by utilizing IF we burn fat and subsequently lose weight.

Many people feel that their metabolism is slow or unstable. Intermittent fasting can speed up and stabilize overall body metabolism. Physiologically IF reduces the amount of insulin produced by the pancreas and allows blood glucose levels to normalize. Over weeks and months metabolic activities of the body naturally become more balanced, normal and regular.

Intermittent fasting has been shown to reduce the type of white blood cell called monocytes. Monocytes are linked with body inflammation. By decreasing inflammation chronic musculoskeletal pains can be improved.

Cancer cells typically feed on glucose. Blood glucose is high when we snack and eat frequently. Conversely, when we fast intermittently, we burn fat. Since most cancer cells cannot feed on fat cancer risk lessons.

Some studies show that intermittent fasting helps the body to clean out toxins and damaged cells. This cleansing and purification reduces tiredness and sluggishness and helps boost energy.

Fasting, in general, is an age-old process that dates back centuries to many faiths and cultures. Almost everyone can easily engage in intermittent fasting and there are a wide array of health benefits

7-DAYS MEAL PLAN

Intermittent fasting is something that so many people have heard about, but perhaps may not totally understand what it is or how to implement it. Essentially, intermittent fasting is a conscious decision to only eat during certain periods of the day. It's not technically a diet because it doesn't limit what you can eat. However, you do have to be mindful of the types of foods you choose. These meals will have to get you through the rest of the day. Whether you've been intermittent fasting for years or just interested in what it looks like, check out this intermittent fasting meal plan.

Before we begin the intermittent fasting meal plan, it's important to understand that intermittent fasting is different than just regular fasting. While there are a variety of ways that people approach this, usually people follow a 16/8 strategy which involves eating 8 hours a day and fasting for the other 16 hours. However, there are numerous strategies that people may follow. The point is to have a period of time in which a person is not consuming calories and then when they do eat, they avoid processed food and focus on whole food recipes.

Many people choose to skip breakfast or dinner, but the method doesn't necessarily require that you skip meals. You should also recognize that the specific caloric intake may vary based on your body's needs to lose weight. Generally, you should focus on eating meals that include fish, lean meats, whole grains, and plenty of veggies. The idea here is that you'll eat a couple of larger meals, but your caloric intake will actually be lower because you will only be consuming foods within a certain timeframe.

Day 1

Breakfast: Spinach Parmesan Baked Eggs

Lunch: Oven-Crisp Fish Tacos

Dinner: Turkey Burrito Skillet

Snack: Dark Chocolate (suggested two squares)

Day 2

Breakfast: Hummus Breakfast Bowl

Lunch: Baked Lemon Salmon and Asparagus Foil Pack

Dinner: Chicken and Broccoli Stir Fry

Snack: Boiled egg

Day 3

Breakfast: 4-Ingredient Protein Pancakes

Lunch: Wild Cod with Moroccan Couscous

Dinner: Honey Garlic Shrimp Stir Fry

Snack: Almonds (suggested 12-14)

Day 4

Breakfast: Ham and Egg Breakfast Cups

Lunch: Sweet Potato and Turkey Skillet

Dinner: Savory Lemon White Fish Fillets

Snack: Two stalks of celery with peanut butter

Day 5

Breakfast: No-Bake Oatmeal Raisin Energy Bites

Lunch: Cucumber Quinoa Salad with Ground Turkey, Olives, Feta

Dinner: Skinny Salmon, Kale, and Cashew Bowl

Snack: 1 cup fresh strawberries

Day 6

Breakfast: Creamy Green Smoothie with a Hint of Mint

Lunch: Baked Chicken and Vegetable Spring Rolls

Dinner: Skinny Turkey Meatloaf

Snack: Avocado and tomatoes

Day 7

Breakfast: Sweet Potato Breakfast Hash

Lunch: Spicy Black Bean and Shrimp Salad

Dinner: Turkey Sausage with Pepper and Onions

Snack: Two cups of chopped celery and carrots

Ready to try an intermittent fasting meal plan for yourself? Keep in mind, the specifics for your diet will vary based on how many calories you should be taking in for weight loss. You'll need to calculate your required calorie intake in order for a meal plan to be most effective.

INTERMITTENT FASTING FOR WEIGHT LOSS TIPS

There's no doubt about it that more and more people today are using intermittent fasting for weight loss. If you're not sure what intermittent fasting is it's basically when you strategically use periods of fasting to force your body into burning fat as a fuel source. This method of weight loss is highly effective but you have to make sure you're doing it right or else you can actually slow your metabolism.

While you are going through a fasting period you should only be consuming water along with Branched Chain Amino Acids (BCAA) which will help prevent the breakdown of muscle. This may be too intense for some people because you will most likely experience hunger and there will be a high level of discipline necessary for intermittent fasting. Those who are for this type of weight loss claim that they can get results quicker than traditional dieting practices such as calorie restriction.

If you're new to intermittent fasting then it's recommended that you do a trial period of 24 hours to make sure you can continue with doing these for an extended period of time. It's going to be natural to become easily irritable towards people during your fasting day so prepare for the worst. I prefer to have a cheat day prior to the fasting day so I can prepare my body for the fast and also accelerate the results. The massive caloric intake of the cheat day primes my body to burn more fat as a fuel source on the fasting day. Be sure to take your BCAA's throughout the day in

5-10 gram servings like you would in place for regular meals. Eventually after you have successfully completed the 24 hours fasts you can progress to more advanced methods of intermittent fasting such as using multiple ones throughout the week.

Intermittent fasting isn't going to be for everyone but if you're serious about getting some real results then this will definitely boost them. Everyone should still learn the basics of a healthy diet and exercise program. You can definitely workout on your fasting days to enhance the fat loss but it will be extremely difficult for many to muster the energy to do so. Overall just make sure you plan ahead prior to your fasting day as it will be instrumental in your success with the program.

CPSIA information can be obtained
at www.ICGtesting.com
Printed in the USA
LVHW022017220121
677171LV00007B/448

9 781801 442459